# Does This Ponytail Make My Butt Look Big?

## Style and Beauty for Every Woman

By Dana Lam and Emily Couch

*Jennalyn,*
*To being confident*
*and fabulous!*
*Always!*
*xoxo*
*Dana Lam*

www.TotalPublishingAndMedia.com

# Dedication

To my amazing family, this is possible because of their love and support. To my mom and dad for breathing belief in me that I can accomplish anything I desire. To my sister, Danell for always making me laugh.
Most of all thank you to
Henry, Ethan & Harrison
I love you!

---DANA


To Tamara, Without your love and support this wouldn't have been possible. To my mom and dad for always pushing me to accomplish my dreams. To my girlfriends, Holly and Samantha for showing me the ways of the dinosaurs.
I love you all.

---EMILY

# Acknowledgements

We would like to thank everyone who supported us with this endeavor.  Without their collaboration this book would not be possible.

Jeff Hunter, Christine Henke, George Horioka, Jessica Lai Lopez, Krissie Kennedy, Lynn Kostel, Bonnie Tornquist, Liz Harris, Christian Senger and Melinda Swiger.

Two of the most amazing women we know contributed great content to our book on life balancing and organizing.
Bonnie Moehle ~ Life Balancing Coach  bonniemoehle.com
Brenda Spangrud ~ Organizer Extraordinaire  sortedorganizing.com

*Our wonderful photographer for creating a great photo for our back cover, which we assure you was not an easy task.*
Desi Smith ~ DES Photography DESPhotoz.com

"I don't understand how a woman can leave the house without fixing herself up a little—if only out of politeness. And then, you never know, maybe that's the day she has a date with destiny. And it's best to be as pretty as possible for destiny." — **Coco Chanel**

## Introductions: Our Why

I often wonder how some people will dress in another thirty years. My grandfather never saw my grandmother without makeup on. My grandmother would wash her face after he was asleep and she would rise before him to put her face back on. Extreme? Maybe, but I think society has gone too far in the opposite direction. Can we please meet in the middle?

I miss the glamour days of yesterday when people dressed up to travel or go to the theater. Who decided that it was okay to roll out of bed, throw your hair in ponytail, and go out in public? June Clever even cleaned her house all dolled up in a dress.

When my mom went to school, girls couldn't wear pants. They had to be ladylike and wear dresses. I remember when I was a nanny working for a woman attorney and she told me of the unspoken rule at her work. The female associates were to wear skirts to the office; however, once you became a partner, you then had the privilege of wearing pants. I found this both interesting and archaic.

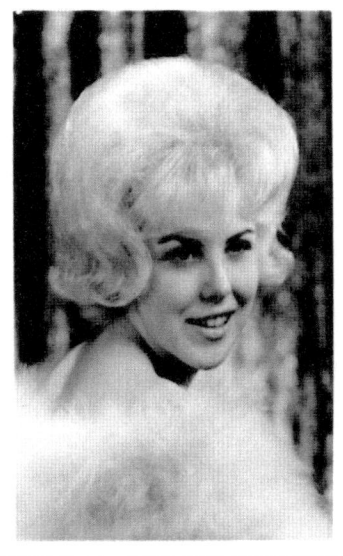

My mom's High School
Graduation Picture

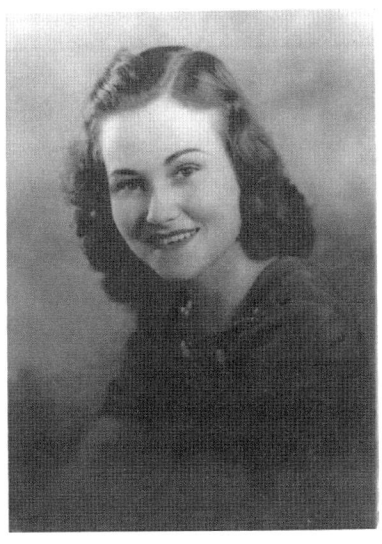

Grandma Glee's High School
Graduation Picture

As for me, I've always loved dresses. Even as a child, dresses were my favorite. I did everything in dresses, even climbing trees. My sister, on the other hand, has always loved pants and still does. I honestly can't remember the last time I've seen her in a skirt or dress. It may have been her wedding. She's a "jeans and t-shirt" kind of girl. Growing up, I would always try to sway her into dressing a little more feminine, and she was so against it. Of course, back then we didn't like each other much, and maybe she just wanted to be the opposite of me. Now, we love each other dearly and wish we could spend more time together. In fact, on a recent trip, we took together with some of her friends and she borrowed some of my clothes. I know she felt great after receiving compliments from her friends. So great that one morning, when I woke up, she was already out and about wearing more of my clothes.

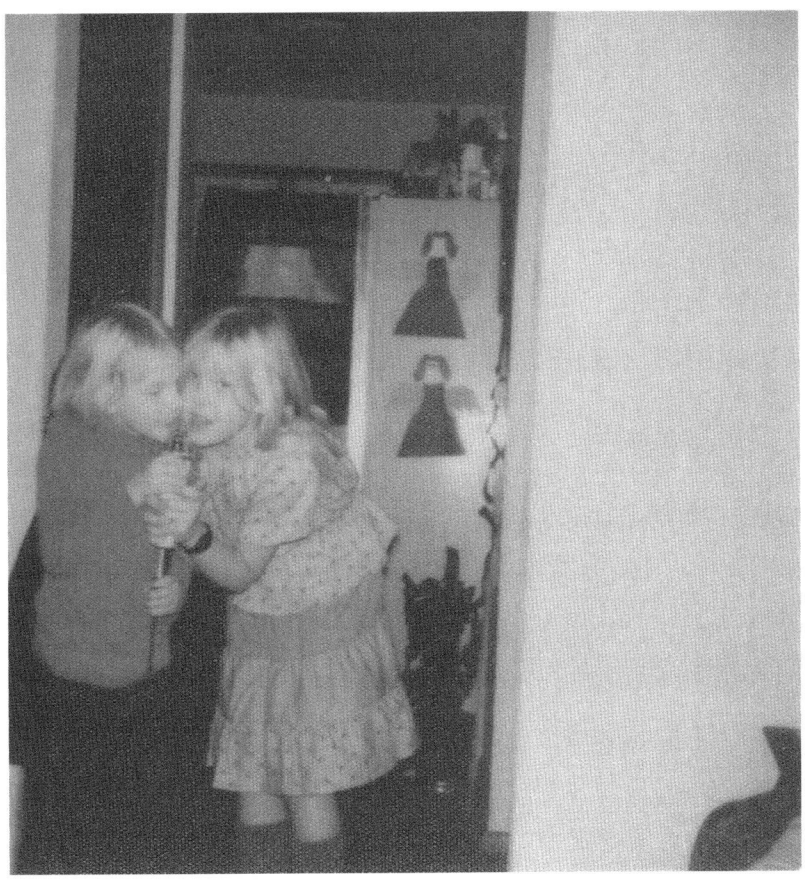

With my sister Danell. As you can see she's wearing pants and I'm in a skirt.

When I was in fourth grade my family moved from Illinois to Arizona and I made a huge fashion faux pas. I thought we had moved to the Wild West and insisted on wearing a cowgirl outfit that I had wore in a singing competition. Oh yes, this outfit had a jean skirt, red plaid shirt with a jean vest and of course cowboy boots. Thankfully I didn't wear the hat. My wonderful mother tried to talk me out of it but I was very insistent.

It was humiliating. I came home in tears vowing to never return again. My mom was very smart. She encouraged me to go to school and hold my head up high. It didn't matter what anyone else thought. I learned that no matter how insecure I was feeling to pretend that I was confident. Basically fake it till I make it. This did get me through high school and my 20 something years.

Growing up in Cottonwood, AZ in a one stop light town was not very interesting. In fact I used to dream that I was switched at birth and that I actually was a Kennedy or a Vanderbilt. My dad used to say that I had a champagne appetite and beer income which I translated to mean that I had the misfortune of being born to a blue collar beer drinking family. Through the years I came to appreciate my family roots. I'm fortunate to have loving caring parents.

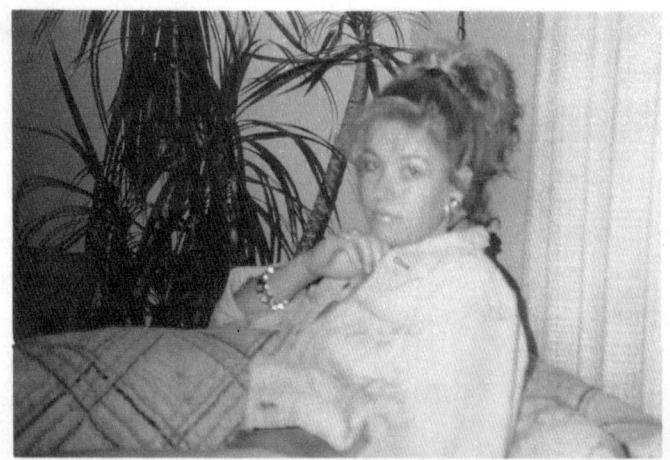

Dana rocking a ponytail in 1986.

Yacht Party in Los Angeles. Dana with her friend Jennifer Murphy, former Miss Oregon and "Apprentice" contestant. From small town to creating the life of my dreams. Anything is possible if you're willing to do what it takes to get there.

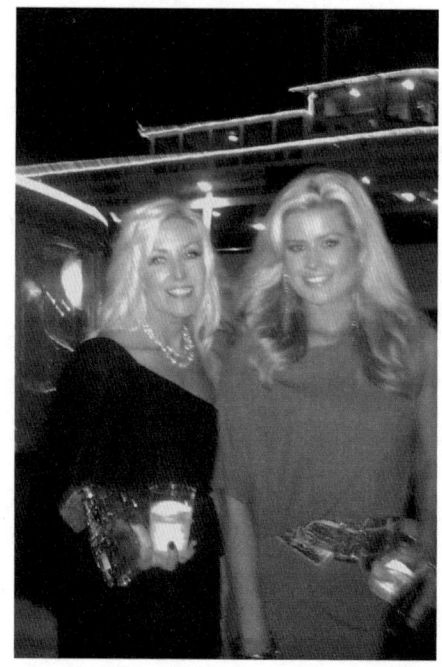

# So how did I end up here?

TEN YEARS AGO, I NEVER WOULD HAVE thought I would be helping people to look and feel wonderful about themselves. My passion at that time, and still is, travel. I worked for American Express for over nine years in the travel division. September of 2001, I was happily married, had one son, and loved my career. I worked in the marketing division for the Fine Hotels & Resorts. I loved my life. Things quickly changed in October of that year. On Halloween, the Phoenix marketing staff was called into a conference room and told over speaker phone that we no longer had jobs. It was a sad day. To top it off, I was dressed like Mia from *Pulp Fiction*. I guess playing dress up is something that I never grew out of.

It was a devastating blow. American Express is an incredible company to work for. The bonus was that I did receive a sixty-day notice and a nearly six-month severance package. Earlier that year, I was invited to a Mary Kay skin care class by my good friend, Angie. Being the supportive friend that I am, I decided to attend. But I wasn't going to buy anything. I honestly thought that Mary Kay was for much older women. And how could products sold out of someone's home be any good, right? So, several hundred dollars later, I left the party a happy Mary Kay customer. After two weeks of using the products, my skin cleared up and I looked amazing. So, after being laid off, and when my beauty consultant Michele told me for the third time how great I would be as an Independent Beauty Consultant, I finally said "yes."

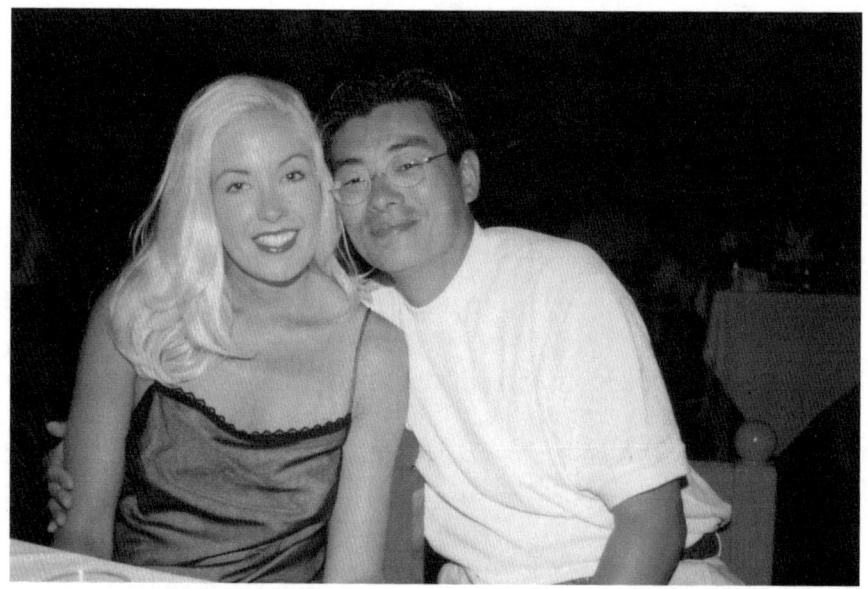

Dana and Henry when they first met

When I broke the news to my husband, he asked if I was going to get a real job, too. I told him it was a real job and that I would own my own business.

I honestly sat on my "assets" for the next six months until my husband suggested that I go back to Corporate America because my severance package was running out. So, I did what any obedient wife would do—I went back to the corporate world. Not really, who could do that after working for themselves? I had a great career, but working for me was so much better, and I loved being at home with my then two-year-old son, Ethan. My husband Henry's comment actually lit a fire inside of me. I thought, *Oh, yeah, I'll show you.* So, the next month, I went on target for my first free car in Mary Kay. Can you believe it only took me a month deciding to get the car? I began my Mary Kay career in December of 2001, and, by that same month, I earned my first free car—a shiny red Grand AM.

TWO MONTHS LATER, I BECAME A SALES DIRECTOR WITH MARY KAY. ONLY TWO PERCENT OF THE SALES FORCE ARE DIRECTORS, SO THIS IS QUITE AN ACCOMPLISHMENT.

In 2007, I earned my second free car, a silver Grand Prix, and became a senior sales director in the company.

In my nearly ten-year career with Mary Kay Cosmetics, I worked with over 1,200 people. Most of them women. A common theme I've heard is "I would love to look like you but I don't have time or money." This would always make me sad to hear and I would try to give the women I worked with ideas for saving time and money. I've heard some crazy things and you'll read more about that in the chapter on skin care and makeup.

My husband and I would both love to live in New York City, but we haven't made that happen yet. So, during the summer of 2009, I convinced my husband to rent an apartment in Manhattan for a month, so our family could test it out. It was fabulous, and, for the month, I created a blog of our family trip so friends and family could see what we were up to. I enjoyed it so much that I realized that I wanted to create a beauty blog to help women. My friend, Brenda, and I were chatting about it one day and she suggested calling the blog "Does This Ponytail Make My Butt Look Big?" making fun a little bit of moms who wear sweats and a ponytail every day.

I loved the name and it stuck. When I started passing out my cards, the strangest thing happened. Women started asking me if I could help them in their closet and with shopping. After saying "no" so many times, I finally said "yes." I wasn't sure I could help someone who was of a different size, age, or shape than me. But quickly, I realized that I found my calling. My life's purpose is to uplift and spark confidence in others. I was able to do this with my image consulting. When a woman looks great on the outside, she feels better on the inside. She exudes confidence.

The goal of my business was to help everyday women. Women like me who are busy wives and mothers. I wanted to be affordable for everyone, so I developed a do-it-yourself course called "5 Weeks to Fabulous" and had rave reviews from my clients who were able to use my tools to get out of their ruts and feel fabulous again. This book was inspired from that class.

So, you may be wondering, "Where does Emily fit into all of this?" I was introduced to her and instantly adored her. She is a fellow fashionista and one of the funniest people I know. She is a brilliant writer, and, if you must know, I originally spoke to her about ghostwriting this book. After speaking to Emily, we realized that it doesn't matter how old you are or where you are in life, we can all easily fall into a fashion rut. Emily is single, young, brunette, and has no kids—the complete opposite of me. We quickly realized that we must do this book together as we can relate to all women.

## SO HERE IS EMILY'S STORY.

# I'VE NEVER UNDERSTOOD MOM JEANS. Even as a child, I would wonder why women would leave their houses looking frumpy.

Frumpiness was never an option for me. When I was young, I was much more into fashion and style than I was playing outside or just being a kid. Whenever I received an invitation to a birthday party, I would spend hours planning the perfect outfit. It wasn't normal behavior for a child. I swear, I was a gay guy at the age of five. My mom has a fabulous story about me in diapers, walking up to the television, pleading with her not to change the channel because Madonna was performing. I said while staring at the television, "Madonna, I just have to touch her." You'll have to ask her about the entire story because it's a total crack up when she tells it. Upon hearing that story about myself, my personality made much more sense to me, and it will to you as well upon reading this book.

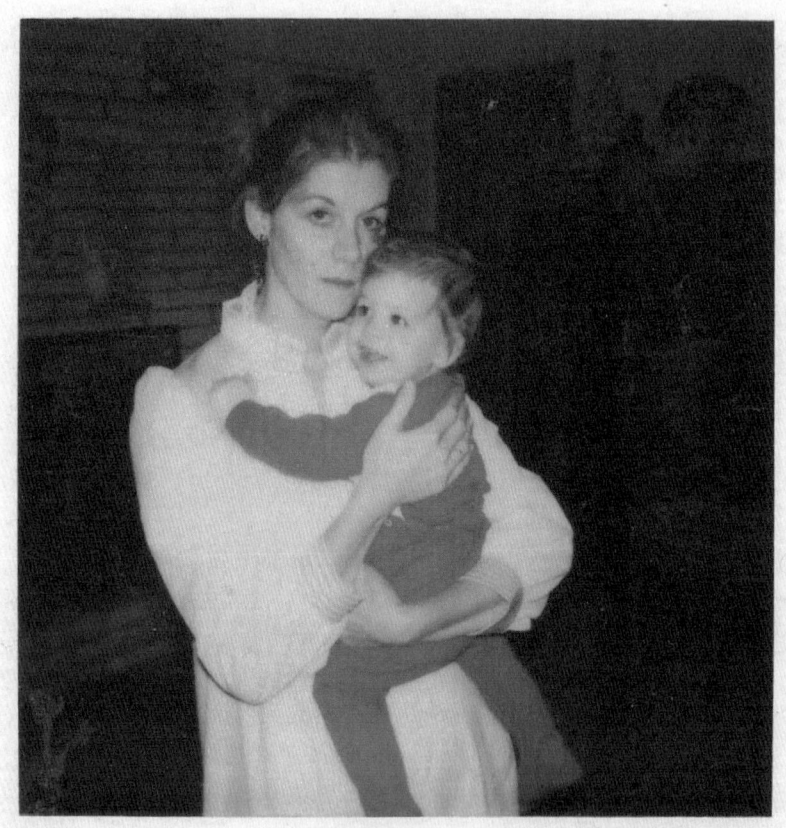

Emily, with her mother. This is one of her favorite pictures.

**Never wanting** to blend in, I made some bold fashion choices. Lycra neon pink stirrup pants and a New Kids on the Block sweater, accompanied by patent leather ballet flats and a massive mop of crimped black hair, made me the envy of every girl in the third grade. (I would totally wear that outfit today if I had access to an NKOTB sweater in my size). While I follow the trends, I tend to stick to what makes me look and feel the most fabulous. In middle school, my favorite outfit consisted of a black body suit, covered with a delightful floral pattern, a faux pearl choker, and black Mary Jane's. In my first day of high school, I wore my favorite outfit circa 1998. Chocolate brown flared corduroys, a tan, fit, V-neck baby tee, and brown high-heeled clogs.

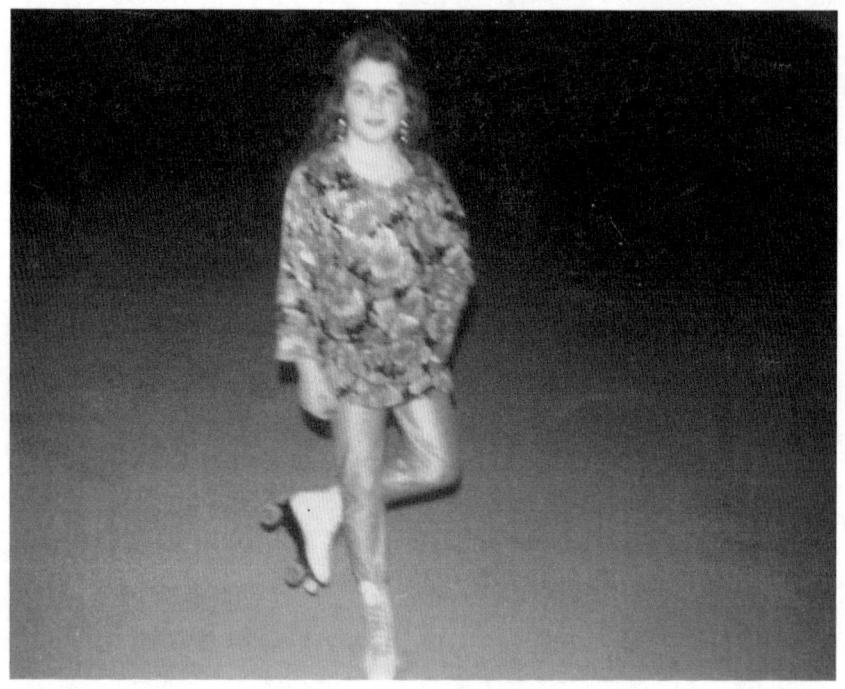

Emily with her pink stretchy pants roller skating on one leg.
That's talent, people.

High school was when I really started to let my style light shine. I loved to cruise the mall but realized that without a job and parents who ironically didn't have access to an unlimited bank account, I couldn't afford to keep up with the proverbial joneses.

Freshman year of high school Emily was asked to the senior prom. Not being able to find a dress she liked she finally found a suitable solution…wearing the dress backward.

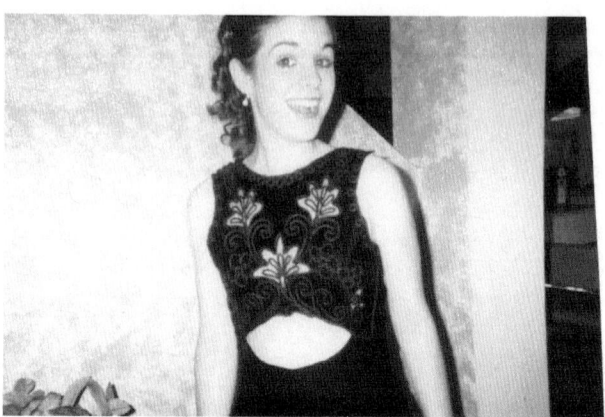

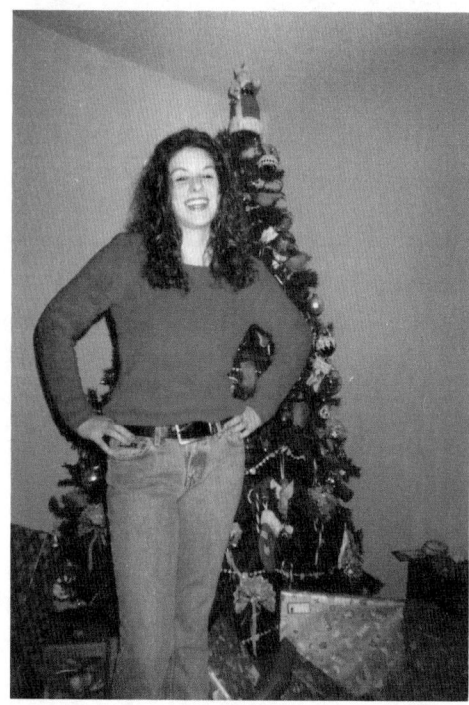

Emily in Arizona Brand Jeans, everyone makes mistakes.

As a child, my mother would take us to consignment shops to buy our clothes because, let's face it, children grow like weeds. And with a father who was sick and with my mother being the sole breadwinner for our family, it was more economical for her to buy our clothes at thrift stores. I used to browse the racks finding the most fabulous garments and made up stories about who donated them. Garage sales were another major source of great fashion finds for me. Once, when I was about seven, I was with my mother's best friend's daughter, Julie, and we decided to spend our allowance at the garage sale next door. I was extremely excited about this garage sale because the neighbor's daughter had impeccable style, and I was waiting for her to grow out of this little black and pink zebra print skirt that had shorts attached. Alas, it was there! But Julie spied it as well and we both went for it. After some mild yelling, a denouncement of a friendship, and take backs of previous Malibu Barbie for Pound Puppy (with three puppies inside) tradesies, the skirt was mine. After my mom caught wind of what happened, she made me give it to Julie, but for the short thirty minutes, it was in my possession. I was the happiest seven-year-old on the planet (and I still think that call on my mom's behalf was total crap).

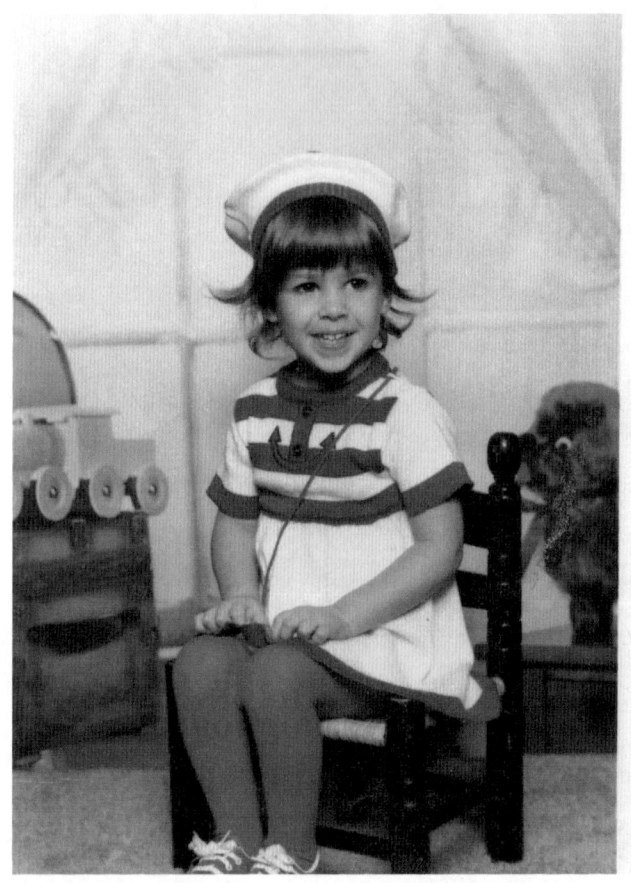

Emily, at the age of 4 having a maritime moment.

**CLOTHES HAVE ALWAYS MADE ME HAPPY.** I can attribute most of my personal development to the foundation of finding my style. Style says who you are, what you're into, and how you live your life. First impressions are everything and it's not something you can get do overs on. Knowing this can help you to begin to dust off those cheese puff covered sweatpants and take your hair out of the ponytail you've been wearing since 1982. Style empowers you. Style can take you on a journey. Style defines my very existence. Let's be clear though, I'm not talking about fashion. Fashion is fleeting, in the moment, dramatic and fantastic. Style is eternal. Style is a timeless way to show the world who you are and can be determining factors in a lot of your major life choices.

I don't work in the style industry like Dana does, but I knew right away that she was someone I wanted to work with. The first time we met, we clicked. We were like two teenage girls in the middle of a professional networking meeting. Immediately, I knew that Dana's style was timeless. The girl knows how to dress and I love style and fashion, so it was a flawless transition. Enough about me, let's get to the good stuff.

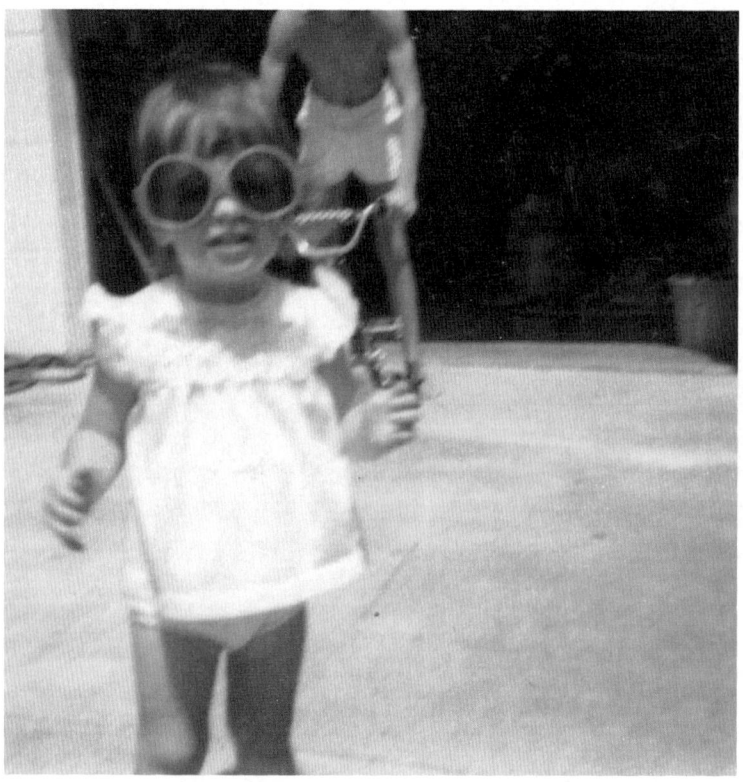

Emily with her first pair of sunnies.

## Why Should You Care?

**How you dress shows how you respect the people around you and yourself.** Let's face it, would you want to run into your ex-boyfriend donning the sweatpants he left at your place six years ago? Our guess is, probably not. So, why would you go out in public dressed like a slob? This shows everyone around you that you don't have any respect for yourself or their visual space. We all like an esthetically pleasing environment. Please don't ruin our view of the hot guy parade with your horrific display of pajamas in public. Let's learn from Emily's mistake, shall we?

"**Like most women**, I was at the bitter end of a broken relationship and was moving on to bigger and better things. I was dating a guy for two years when I was offered an amazing position in another city on the other side of the country. We had a hard decision to make and we ultimately decided to call it quits. On the morning of my flight, I was less than thrilled, could not stop from crying, and prepared for the worst. My motto is to look fabulous and everything else will fall into place…today was the exception. I threw my hair up in a messy bun (not the acceptable version). This was my first mistake. All of my clothes were packed and I didn't have the energy to rifle through them, so I grabbed an oversized navy blue tank top and a pair of distressed white skinny jeans. This was my second mistake. I also decided that wearing flip-flops was acceptable in the airport. This was my biggest mistake. You can't run in flip-flops. My makeup was smeared as I hugged my ex goodbye and prepared for my flight that was delivering me into my new life. As I was walking toward my gate, I spotted none other than my ex-fiancé and his new wife. Shocked and obviously still rattled from my sorrowful good-bye, I froze, hoping that somehow I would become invisible. This did not work. He spotted me almost immediately and made his way over. I had envisioned this moment a million times in my mind and this was most definitely not how it was supposed to play out. I was not wearing the "make him wish he never dumped me" outfit. This consisted of the metallic gold Louboutins I spotted last year, that little black dress with sleeves and had the back cut out that I saw in a shop at that one place in Miami, and, of course, a huge engagement ring that I clearly did not have in my possession. I was supposed to be flawless, and this was not ideal. This was happening. CODE RED! I clearly didn't have time to work on any of the

## NA'S STORY

When I was a
freshman in high
school, I was
completely
infatuated with a
senior. Let's call
him Laurance to
protect the
innocent.

He would not give me the time of day. So, fast forward, ten years later, I'm in a tanning salon and Laurance was there and he looks better than ever, I could hardly breathe. He went in and I whispered to the girl at the front desk, "Is his name Laurance?" She nodded "yes." So, for the whole twenty minutes, I was horizontal in the tanning bed. I was remembering high school and thinking about how hot he looks. I also wondering if he still recognized me. As I'm leaving the salon, he had been waiting for me outside and struck up a conversation. I let the conversation go on for a while and then brought up our high school. He stated that there was no way we went to high school together as he would have remembered me. So, I told him sorry and that he had his chance and I was now in a relationship. Thankfully, I looked amazing. I have long, blonde, wavy hair. My makeup is done just right. I'm in great shape and have a fabulous ivory tank dress and some cute sandals on. This day could have played out much differently. What if I had my hair in a ponytail, no makeup on, and been dressed like a slob? I know for a fact that Laurance wouldn't have been waiting for me. What would have been going through my mind? When I left the salon, I would have been thinking crazy things. Maybe that Laurance had remembered me and was thankful he never went out with me. I would have left deflated. Fortunately, for me, I left feeling amazing and had the satisfaction that someone had their chance and didn't take it and he missed out."

previous statements, so I just did what any girl wo
situation. I claimed to be running late for my flight.
my face from seeing him could totally pass for the pa
a flight, right? I bowed out less than gracefully and
power walk in my flip-flops to the end of the termin
entire way. A few weeks later, I received an e-mail
from him, asking if I was okay. I disregarded and mov

# What can we learn this? Looking good your confidence!

Lacking confidence in that situation was not b
anyone, but possibly his new wife. I'm sure she
the fact that Emily looked like she had just ro
bed. Emily was not thrilled. In fact, Emily had
would have taken the extra effort that morning.
is the key to success, so why not start with makii
look good on the outside? **When you look b
the outside, you feel better on the ir**
aren't saying that beauty and fashion are t
confidence and success. We are saying it's
excellent way to kick start the path to a more
you. Why not be the best "you" you can be?
confident, and original.

## DANA'S STORY

"When I was a freshman in high school, I was completely infatuated with a senior. Let's call him Laurance to protect the innocent.

He would not give me the time of day. So, fast forward, ten years later, I'm in a tanning salon and Laurance was there and he looks better than ever, I could hardly breathe. He went in and I whispered to the girl at the front desk, "Is his name Laurance?" She nodded "yes." So, for the whole twenty minutes, I was horizontal in the tanning bed. I was remembering high school and thinking about how hot he looks. I was also wondering if he still recognized me. As I'm leaving the salon, he had been waiting for me outside and struck up a conversation. I let the conversation go on for a while and then brought up our high school. He stated that there was no way we went to high school together as he would have remembered me. Alas, I told him sorry and that he had his chance and I was now in a relationship. Thankfully, I looked amazing. I have long, blonde, curly hair. My makeup is done just right. I'm in great shape and have a fabulous ivory tank dress and some cute sandals on. This story could have played out much differently. What if I had my hair in a ponytail, no makeup on, and been dressed like a slob? I know for a fact that Laurance wouldn't have been waiting for me. What would have been going through my mind? When I left the salon, I would have been thinking crazy things. Maybe that Laurance had remembered me and was thankful he never went out with me. I would have left deflated. Fortunately, for me, I left feeling amazing and had the satisfaction that someone had their chance and didn't take it and he missed out."

previous statements, so I just did what any girl would do in this situation. I claimed to be running late for my flight. The panic on my face from seeing him could totally pass for the panic of missing a flight, right? I bowed out less than gracefully and proceeded to power walk in my flip-flops to the end of the terminal, crying the entire way. A few weeks later, I received an e-mail via Facebook from him, asking if I was okay. I disregarded and moved on."

# What can we learn from this? Looking good builds your confidence!

Lacking confidence in that situation was not beneficial to anyone, but possibly his new wife. I'm sure she relished in the fact that Emily looked like she had just rolled out of bed. Emily was not thrilled. In fact, Emily had wished she would have taken the extra effort that morning. Confidence is the key to success, so why not start with making yourself look good on the outside? **When you look better on the outside, you feel better on the inside.** We aren't saying that beauty and fashion are the key to confidence and success. We are saying it's a really excellent way to kick start the path to a more confident you. Why not be the best "you" you can be? Be sexy, confident, and original.

## THE GOAL

# WE WANT OUR CLOTHES to make us look fabulous, shapely, and confident.

We strive to express ourselves through how we dress. Express the most powerful you. The goal is not to be vain, but to be confident with what you're portraying to the world. If you wear the right clothes, you can enhance the parts of your body that work for you and hide the parts that you don't love. You should develop a loving relationship with yourself. The ultimate goal is for your external image to embrace your internal fabulousness.

# The

# Lies

# and

# Excuses

# Fashion magazines are your bible:

# LIE

Fashion magazines are the enemy. They are meant to sell ads not promote your most fabulous self. First off, the average woman cannot afford a $1,000 belt. They lie to us and make us believe that without this season's "it" accessory, you're not fashionable or fabulous. LIES! Secondly, nobody can live up to the model standards in said fashion magazines. We are not a size 0 and we don't believe you have to be a size 0 to be confident, fabulous, and sexy. We like carbs, cocktails, and cupcakes and don't plan on giving any of those up.

*"People should be fashion conscious not fashion victims"*
*~ Randi Rahm, fashion designer*

# Style is effortless:

# LIE

Effortless style is a fantasy, it takes work. Do you think that Nicole Richie rolls out of bed looking Bohemian chic? The answer is "no." Most likely, (and we are just guessing) she has a team of stylist that make sure every hair is just messy enough to encompass her personal style. We aren't saying that you should out and hire a team of stylist (unless you want to hire us, then go for it), we are just saying that you should take the time to create your own style. If you don't take the time, the time will take you.

"The only rule is don't be boring and dress cute wherever you go. Life is too short to blend in"
~ Paris Hilton

# To look great you must look like a model:

# LIE

Please reread point 1 and allow us to expand upon it. We are not models. In fact, we aren't even close. We take good care of ourselves but we won't end up on a runway anytime soon. Don't feed into the lies that society tells you. Embrace the body you have and dress to enhance what you've been given. There is a fashionable solution for every body type.

"Embrace your own personal beauty—love who you are today and everyday."
~ Robert Jones

# I don't have the time to mess with my appearance:

# LIE

Seriously, this is the most ridiculous statement we have ever heard. You take a shower every morning, right? (We hope so.) You get dressed every morning, right? Why not dress to impress?

"There are no ugly women, only lazy ones."
~ Helena Rubinstein

# I can't afford a new wardrobe:

# LIE

Consign. Consign. Consign. We cannot stress this enough. Fashion does not have to be expensive. Sarah Jessica Parker said, "Fashion is not a luxury," and we couldn't agree more. Once you're sick of something in your closet, take it to a local consignment shop and trade it in. This is a relatively inexpensive way to build your wardrobe without breaking the bank. NEVER go in debt for fashion. You will resent the clothes in your closet and they will no longer inspire your confidence and make you feel amazing. Who wants a constant reminder of their lingering credit card bill?

"*I like my money right where I can see it...hanging in my closet*"
~ Carrie Bradshaw, Sex and The City

# I need to lose weight:

# LIE

Maybe you do and maybe you don't, but you have to dress to fit your body NOW. Nothing is a bigger motivator to get into shape than looking and feeling great. Dana always says, "Dress for who you are now, not five pounds from now." We all have a pair of jeans we purchased as "motivation" that sit in our closet as a daily reminder of our weight loss failure. Consign those jeans and buy a pair that makes you look fabulous NOW. When you lose the weight, then you can go buy a fabulous pair of jeans that are a size smaller as a reward. While you're at it, get a massage. Those always help us feel fabulous.

"In all likelihood, you don't need to diet. You just need a different silhouette and size."
~ Rachel Zoe

# I don't need to look good everyday:

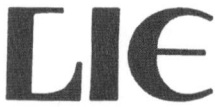

Do you need to feel good everyday?

You should dress everyday as if you may run into the love of your life that broke your heart. Need we say more?

## Let's Get Started

# WE KNOW THAT TAKING ON THE TASK OF ORGANIZING YOUR CLOSET IS DAUNTING AND CAN BE SCARY.

**Relax,** this should be a fun experience. Do you know that most people only wear ten to twenty percent of what's in their closet?

**Keeping that in mind, pick out the things in your closet that you know you want to keep.**

Keeping that in mind, pick out the things in your closet that you know you want to keep. It should be easy to identify the staples you wear on a daily basis. This eliminates ten to twenty percent of your organizational woes. Ask yourself what image you want to project in all aspects of your life. What is your career, social, casual and formal style identity? What celebrity style do you covet the most? Out of your friends, who do you think dresses the cutest? Figure out what you like and strive for it. If you're not sure what your style is, the best way to figure this out is to look online, visit malls frequently, and take a mental picture of people you see out and about who look fabulous. Elvis said, "Imitation is the sincerest form of flattery." Don't be scared to ask people where they shop.

## When Is the Last Time You Put Effort into Your Appearance?

Think of a time when you put effort into your appearance. How much energy do you put into getting ready for a special occasion, date night, job interview, or important business meeting? Did you not feel great? You should put this amount of passion into your everyday routine. Think about when you were a teenager. Remember how much time it took just to get ready to go to the mall? Tone that down a bit, add a martini, and apply that to your adult life.

There is no need to go overboard with your daily routine like you did when you were a teenager, just take some more time to pamper your appearance. We promise it will make a huge difference. We always deserve to feel that great. We strive to feel as fabulous as we did the night we felt and looked our greatest. Make that same amount of effort every single day and get prepared to feel the confidence oozing from your pores. It's a fabulous feeling and it will turn heads.

## What's In Your Closet?

When you open your closet, do stare blankly, and scream, "I have nothing to wear!?" If you can, put down this book, go to the mirror, and answer a few questions. How do you feel about yourself right now? Do you like your outfit? Do you feel confident and beautiful? Are you dressed how you want to be dressed for public interaction?

You may not feel very good about yourself right now, which is probably why you bought our book. Hold tight, we are going to help you fix this little problem. Do us a favor: pull out your favorite outfit, put it on. How do you feel now? Confident, sexy, and beautiful? What if all of your clothes made you feel this way?

## Fashion Is Personal:

**Do us a favor: try not to follow trends. The latest trends may not always look good on you. The key to confidence is looking good and feeling good. If you don't look good in the latest fashion trend, then leave it on the runway. Take harem pants. Nobody looked good in harem pants, yet everyone wore them. Personally, we didn't get it. The media, celebs, and fashion magazines determine the trends, but we don't always agree with their choices. For example, Dana looks fabulous in capri pants while Emily can't pull off the look (which irritates her). Find a look you love and feel fabulous in and stick with it (with the exception of harem pants). Who cares if it's not the "hot new look" of the season. If you look great in the look you love, you feel great. And people will notice that automatically, thinking you're the "hot new thing." Leave the harem paints where they belong—with Sienna Miller and Princess Jasmine.**

## Have You Been Stuck In a Time Warp?

When is the last time you went shopping for new clothes? If you can't remember, it's probably time to clean out the old closet.

**If you haven't worn something in over a year, toss it.**

If you've had a garment for over two years, burn it. Don't get stuck in a time warp and don't be afraid to update your look. If you can't afford to go out and purchase a new look, try consigning and thrift shopping. We are huge fans of both. If you're over the age of twenty and still wearing the same styles and clothes that you did in high school, you need to follow our advice. This same message applies to college graduates. If you graduated over a year ago and you're still rocking your sorority letters across the back of your sweats or on your chest, put down this book and immediately go and clean out your closet. Don't make us come down there!

## Shopping Takes Practice and Work:

**Shopping should be fun, but we've talked to several clients who hate shopping because they've built a box around themselves. They only try on certain colors or styles. They only shop at discount stores, among the sales racks, or online.** So, when they receive their clothes, they are ill-fitting or not what they expected. That is a major cause of anxiety or frustration.

## Never Shop on Price Alone

Okay, so first, hear us out on this. We love a great deal just as much as the next person. Finding that beautiful white leather St. John coat for ninety percent off made Dana's day. She loved the coat before she knew what a great deal it was. What we are trying to say is that you're better off purchasing fewer items that you love than purchasing items that are okay just because they are a bargain.

We recommend that when you're out shopping, you select items to try on without looking at their tags. You don't need to know how much it is right now. Just focus on items that catch your eyes. As you're trying on, you'll have two piles: one for the items you like and another for items you don't. When you're done trying items on, you will then review the items you like and decide which ones you liked the most. Now, you can look at the price of each item. You may also want to take the items to a price scanner in the store or to a cashier to verify if any of the items are on sale. So, when deciding which items to purchase, take the amount of money you've budgeted and be sure to stay within that when making your selections.

> Never go into debt for fashion. Purchase the best quality products that you can afford.

We recently went shopping with a client who only shopped on sale. This resulted in her having a closet full of clothes that weren't fabulous. She didn't love them nor did she feel fabulous in them. We went shopping and her instructions were to not look at the price tags. She decided to purchase everything she tried on that day that she loved. When we were checking out, she said she couldn't believe she was going to purchase a blouse for $89. She usually would not have even tried on an item at that price. However, she loved the way this blouse made her feel. It fit her great and was the perfect color for her skin tone. To her delight, the blouse was on sale for only $19. It just wasn't marked on the tag. This scenario was repeated for several of the items. She was elated and will never shop the way she used to.

**So, remember to shop for how items look and make you feel and not based on price.**

If you have a pair of pants that were okay and a great deal at $10 but you only wear them once, is it that a good deal? What about a pair of amazing pants that fit you great that you purchase for $100 and wear all the time because they go with everything? So if you wear them twenty times that's only $5 per wear. Which is a better deal?

# Determining Your Style

**Define Your Style:** You have to figure out who you are and what you're trying to say to the world. How do you want people to see you? Define what color palette works best for you. Define which pieces in your closet help you feel beautiful and which pieces inspire confidence and passion. This will help you define who you are and what your personal style is.

## DANA'S STORY OF HER PERSONAL STYLE.

Your style may change through the years as mine has. In high school, I always wanted to be different. I never wanted to look like anyone else. The unique dressing and hairstyles continued into my early twenties, and then I went completely opposite and started dressing classic. Then in my mid to late twenties, I loved dressing more like Jackie O. and the '60s chic. Now that I'm over forty, I'm definitely more classic/chic in how I dress. However, some days, I like to be more whimsical and flirty. I'm evolving. So every year I evaluate what is the image I want to project to the world. Sometimes we get so busy that we lose our identity and we just go with the flow. And that's how you get stuck in a rut. Being aware when you're on the path of falling into a rut is key.

**Sometimes** fitting into a defined box isn't for you. Emily is all over the map when it comes to defining herself as it pertains for style.

One day, she is Bohemian and whimsical, and the next day, she's classical and refined. You might fall under this category and that's okay. You might have a different daytime style than an evening style. Buttoned up, office style during the day and wild, flirty party girl at night. You don't have to stick to one style. You can join Emily and label yourself a stylistic free spirit. That's a book all it's own. Regardless, if you're able to define your style or prefer to be a free spirit, pay attention this week to window displays, people on the street, and reviews of stores and designers online. By simply paying a tad more attention to the fashion and style around you, it can open your eyes to new and exciting styles. Remember to be true to yourself above all else and your personality will shine through you.

# Purging Your Wardrobe

## The Goal—

We want our clothes to help us feel fabulous, shapely, and confident. We live by the motto "fake it till you make it." We know that wearing the right clothing is a huge source of confidence for women. You will hear us say this many times throughout this book, when you look great, you feel great. We want you to express the most powerful "you" that you can be. Let us take the stress out of getting ready. Translation: let's unclutter your closet. We want you to be able to wear everything in your closet. But more importantly, we want you to love everything in your closet. This is going to save you time and money. You're going to train your brain to shop for what you love and what you know you're actually going to wear, instead of shopping for price or convenience. Believe it or not, people really do shop for clothes factoring only in convenience. If you choose to limit yourself to only a few stores, you're only hurting yourself. Price can be a more limiting factor than convenience, so hear us out. We love Stacy London from the television show *What Not to Wear*. She's super spunky. We like spunky. We appreciate spunky. She said something to a client that

> You will hear us say this many times throughout this book, *when you look great, you feel great.* We want you to express the most powerful "you" that you can be.

65

has stuck with us for years: "If you wouldn't buy it at full price, then don't buy it when it's on sale." That statement officially made us rethink the way we were shopping. Several of our clients were only shopping in the clearance section or limiting the amount of money they were willing to spend on each garment. What is the outcome of this? You end up with a closet full of clothes that you don't love. We want to love every single piece in our closet. We want to know that when we go to our closet in the morning, we will be able to put together an outfit we will love with a minimal amount of time and stress. You should still shop in the clearance section, just don't limit yourself to ONLY shop in that section. **We have learned that we would rather walk away from a store with one garment we love than ten we just kind of like. Make sense? Okay, let's get to your closet. Are you ready?**

## Where to Start—

AS WE STATED earlier, most people only wear ten to twenty percent of what's in their closet. We know this is true because Emily recently cleaned out her closet and got rid of eighty percent. So, clearly our calculations must be accurate. She consigned most of it. And what she couldn't consign, she donated to Goodwill. Consigning is awesome because you can make money to buy new clothes that you look and feel fabulous in. It's been our experience that, at most, consignment shops will offer you forty percent cash and fifty percent in store credit after they have sold your garment. Be careful with the extra ten percent that you're offered to use as credit in store. Ten percent (or whatever percentage they offer you for in store credit) isn't worth it if you can't find something you love. Donating has its own rewarding benefits—tax write-offs and the warm fuzzies you get from being philanthropic. Philanthropy is sexy and makes us feel confident. We like helping others, hence, the reason for this book.

Okay…it's go time.

Time to organize!

# Create five categories

1. Toss

2. Donate

3. Consign

4. Keep

5. Tailor

**Things to consider:**

**Do you love it?**

**Is it flattering?**

**Does it project the image you want the world to see?**

**Hold up each item,** you will either say, "I like this" or "I don't like this." If you know by looking at the item that you're not going to keep it, then don't try it on. If you believe that you do like it, then go ahead and try it on.

# Be Aware of the Four Wardrobes

# Professional

# Social

# Casual

# Formal

# THINGS TO CONSIDER:

- Does it fit me or can it be altered to fit me?
- Will I spend the extra money to alter it?
- Is it flattering on?
- Do the colors go well with your skin tone? Does it make you look shapely?
- Does it hide or flatter any problem areas you may have? Do you feel fabulous?
- Is it age appropriate?

If you answer "yes" to ALL of these questions, then proceed.

Review: Does it project the image you want the world to see? Is it a casual piece for going out with friends? Is it a piece you would wear on date? Is that how you'd want someone you were trying to impress to view you? Is this a work piece? Does this piece portray business or pleasure? Can you be taken seriously in the office wearing this garment?

**Does this garment fit you now, not who you are five pounds from now? If it doesn't fit and can't be altered, then toss it.**

Ultimately, to keep this garment, you must answer "yes" to these three questions:

## DO YOU LOVE IT?
## IS IT FLATTERING?
## DOES IT PROJECT THE IMAGE YOU WANT THE WORLD TO SEE?

## This is what stays in your closet.

**Even if a garment is something brand new or stylish and looks good on other people but not on you, that's okay. Just get rid of it. It's not serving your better interest. We promise, you'll feel better. Also, don't keep anything you haven't worn in the past year.**

If you find that you're always procrastinating de-cluttering, an easy fix is to turn all of your hangers backwards. When you wear an item, put it back in the closet with the hangers as you normally would. Note your calendar to review your closet six months from now. You can toss any of the hangers that are still backwards because you obviously haven't worn the item. Obviously, you want to do this seasonally for the items.

**Letting go of items that no longer serve you will open up your closet and your life to new and better things.**

**Toss:** This is reserved for the clothing that simply gets thrown or made into rags for cleaning around the house.

**Toss** anything that is worn so badly that you wouldn't even consider wearing it to play in the dirt. Anything with worn-out elastic, holes, or stains are a given. Undergarments, socks, and bathing suits are among the items that should be tossed as well, yuck. Shoes that aren't in good condition, like your old running shoes that are duct taped together, or a pair of plastic flip-flops that have seen better days should be tossed as well.

**Donate:** Please donate anything that another person may find useful.

# Consign: Our favorite section

You can consign items that are usually four years old or less. They must be pressed and on hangers when you take them in.

The reason for this is that the garments will look much more presentable. Make sure they're in new or like new condition. If they're new, make sure you leave the tags on, so the value of the garment is obvious. This will lead to more money in your pocket.

Research the consignment stores in your area and try to get referrals from friends. Make sure to call ahead for their consignment hours. Most consignment stores will only take incoming garments during certain days and hours. Remember to ask which season they are taking. Some stores won't take coats, jackets, sweaters, and winter clothing during summer and reversed. There is no sense in hauling bags of sundresses and tank tops to a consignment shop that isn't taking them. Certain stores will purchase your clothes outright and give you cash while others will wait until your items are sold to pay you for them. If they aren't sold, then they are generally donated. Some stores will notify you if an item doesn't sell while others will not, and it's your responsibility to pick through the racks and reclaim your items. The bottom line: ask a ton of questions, know the rules of the store, and keep a copy of your contract.

# Keep: Keep whatever is left.

# Tailor: Only keep things to tailor if you know for sure you will take the time to get it done. If you know it's going to sit in your closet or car for months before you take it to a tailor then just donate it.

# Beyond the Skirts and Blouses.

**Accessories** can make or break an outfit.

## Accessories: Belts, Shoes, Jewelry, Scares, Hair Enhancements

Filter through your accessories like you did your clothing. Let the same questions you asked yourself earlier be your driving force when determining which pile your accessories will ultimately end up.

Random Tidbits of Highly valuable information.

## Sentimental Pieces:

I bet you're asking yourself about those sentimental pieces of clothing that you never wear—the t-shirt from college or the dress you were wearing when you met your husband. Are you still wearing those garments? Probably not. And if they don't fit, they are just sitting in a closet or dresser taking up space. You're going to continue to shuffle past them for years to come, and then eventually toss them. If you can stomach it, just toss them. It will be refreshing. Make room in your closet for new memories while fondly remembering the old ones. If you can't toss them, put them in a beautiful box out of the way. It doesn't need to be in the prime real estate in your closet.

## Costumes:

Okay, these issues always get us laughing. How long have you been holding on to a certain piece of clothing claiming that you're going to be Madonna for Halloween? *Forever*, we are sure of it. Get rid of pieces you're saving for a "just in case" moment to occur. They serve no purpose in your closet and cause added stress when trying to get dressed.

The solution is to keep it with your other Halloween items, again, not in the prime real estate area of your closet.

NOW THAT YOU'VE ORGANIZED YOUR CLOTHES AND CLEANED OUT YOUR CLOSET, TAKE STOCK IN WHAT YOU HAVE LEFT.

**What color dominates your closet? How many casual, career, social, and dressy pieces do you have? You can now determine what is missing to get ready for the next steps. We promise, when this is over, you will have a feeling of accomplishment and relief. Clutter or hanging on to things that don't serve your better purpose is stifling to your growth.**

## CAN WEARING PRETTY LINGERIE MAKE YOU FEEL MORE CONFIDENT?

## Dana's story

> I HAVE TO SAY THAT
> I'VE GONE THROUGH
> DIFFERENT PHASES IN
> MY LIFE WITH
> REGARDS TO LINGERIE.

In my twenties, my undergarments were amazing. I spent so much money at Victoria's Secret and everything had to match, always. An ex of mine was from Europe and he couldn't believe how inexpensive our lingerie was here in the US. Most European women put a lot of time, money, and thought into their undergarments.

I DO HAVE TO SAY that after being married for many years and being a mom, I allowed both my sleepwear and my lingerie to lose its pizzazz. I don't know why or how this happened. It was slowly over time. As I was packing for a business trip, I realized that I would be embarrassed for anyone to see my less than glamorous boudoir apparel.

The solution was to practice what I preach with my clients. I went through my undergarments and sleepwear and threw away everything that no longer served me. Wow, it was a lot. This forced me to purchase some new items that made me look glamorous and sexy.

*I had forgotten how great I feel lounging around my bedroom in some cute pajamas.*

Here are some things that I discovered from wearing nice lingerie.

1. I feel sexier and more confident just knowing that I'm wearing something nice and pretty.
2. I feel as though I have a secret and that no one else knows what I'm wearing under my clothes.
3. I like wearing it for me. So what if no one else sees it or if my husband doesn't notice it. It makes me feel special and I'm worth it.

We recently stopped at Anastasia's Bath Body Boudoir for our VIP fashion tour, and everyone appreciated the beauty of the store and the beautiful garments. Some of the comments I heard people say were things like "I love this, I just wish I had someone to wear it for," or "I would get this if I had a better body." Ladies, what I would say to that is *dress for yourself and no one else*. Even if you don't have anyone special to show off your garments, there is nothing like being prepared for the future. Love and appreciate the body you're in today.

**We can be our worst critics. Realize that goddesses come in all shapes and sizes.**

## Love Your Skin & Hair

WE'RE SURE YOU KNOW THAT YOUR SKIN IS THE LARGEST ORGAN OF YOUR BODY. YET, SOMETIMES, I THINK WE DON'T GIVE IT MUCH THOUGHT. WE'VE HAD CLIENTS ACTUALLY TELL US THAT THEY USE WHATEVER IS IN THE SHOWER TO WASH THEIR FACE. SHAMPOO? BUTT SOAP? WHAT WE MEAN BY BUTT SOAP IS THAT SOME PEOPLE USE THE BODY SOAP IN THE SHOWER TO WASH THEIR FACE WITH...AND YOU KNOW WHERE THAT SOAP HAS BEEN. YUCK! TO THIS WE REPLY, "WOULD YOU USE TOOTHPASTE UNDER YOUR ARMS OR DEODORANT ON YOUR TEETH?"

It's so important that you use products made for your skin type.

Keep in mind that your skin can change with seasons or with age. You may find that when you were younger, you were oilier, but now you're dry on your cheeks and oily in the T-zone. Or you could be oily in the summer and dry in the winter. So be aware of your skin always.

Your skin starts aging at about twenty, so it's never too soon to start a good skin care routine. We recommend a great cleanser, day moisturizer with spf (the difference between a grape and a raisin—moisture) and an evening moisturizer, eye cream, and an exfoliator like microdermabrasion. This is the bare minimum any women should be using and this won't take a lot of time. Get a cleanser that you can use in the shower.

> Of course, there are a lot of supplemental products you can add for the following:

- Antiaging
- Dark circles
- Puffy eyes
- Toning and tightening
- Smoothing
- Dark spots

NOW, LET'S TALK ABOUT MAKEUP. One of our favorite articles is "Eyeing My Career in a World Without Mascara." Lucy Chabot Reed wrote this article that appeared in the *Washington Business Journal.* Lucy basically didn't feel she needed to wear make up to be taken professionally. She thought that her work should show for itself.   What she discovered is that we are judged by our outward appearance.  If you're not taking time to pay attention to the details on yourself, what other details will you miss when it comes to your career? We hope you will look this article up on the web.

> If you remember Dana's story about her grandmother and how she never let her husband see her without makeup.

We feel at the very minimum that you should put on a little lip gloss and mascara.   That is the very least you can do.   Makeup isn't meant to cover your face but to enhance your natural beauty. Foundation is actually a protection from the environment while it evens your skin tone.

# Even though there is a thirteen-year

difference between us, we were both influenced by *Cindy Crawford's Basic Face*. This is a great book on maximizing your natural beauty.   We hope you will ALWAYS put your best face forward.

## WE WILL BE BRIEF ABOUT HAIR.

We heard someone once said that if you haven't had a compliment on your hair in the past two weeks, you should cut, dye, or buy some more of it.  It's not about the ponytail. But if you wear a ponytail every day, then you may need an intervention.

## Release the Guilt

**IN WORKING WITH WOMEN,** I've found very often that we sometimes have guilt when it comes to spending time and money on ourselves. Well, we want to give you permission to release the guilt. We have our careers and family obligations that use up our resources, and we give so much that there is usually not much left for us. We get the miniscule drops that are left as we fall exhausted into bed each evening, knowing that tomorrow we have to do it all again. We're wives, mothers, daughters, and sisters. We volunteer our time and donate to our causes because it makes us feel valuable and good about ourselves.

Dana was at an event with Bob Proctor as the speaker. He was commending us for attending the event and talking about the excuses we could have made for not being there. He also encouraged us to be at the next event. Something he said really resonated within. He said, "You're going to spend your time and your money somewhere." This applies to so many things. In this instance, you're going to spend your time and money anyway, so why not spend time taking care of yourself? When you take care of yourself, its like recharging your batteries. I promise you'll have more to give back if you take care of yourself first.

**We can hear you now you're probably justifying to yourself that we just don't understand your life. How can you buy new clothes for yourself when your kids need new clothes for school?** Or maybe you just don't have time to go shopping. Because after work, homework, and getting dinner for the family, you wouldn't have much time. I've found that as women, we want something badly enough that we can make anything happen. Do you want to look and feel fabulous? Do want to take care of yourself? Well, guess what? You're the only one who can take care of you. I think we should take advice from flight attendants.

Be sure to put your oxygen mask on first before you help anyone else. You can't help anyone if you're dead.

For us, this includes things like getting manicures, pedicures, massages, facials, having good skin care products, and, of course, taking the time on a regular basis to shop for great clothes. Clothes that we love, that fit, look flattering, and project the image that we want the world to see.

# Be sure to take the time to clean out your

closet at least twice a year, but preferably four times. We sometimes tend to hold onto things that no longer serve us for too long. This task will actually save you time and money. You may not have thought about this, but if you consign items, you can add money to your pocket. When you know what you have, can see everything in your closet, know that you love everything, and that it fits you, it will save you time in getting ready. Also, you won't make purchasing mistakes by buying something you already own but you just can't find in your closet.

The next step is to take the time that you deserve to go shopping on a regular basis. Do you love shopping or loathe it? We've found that you either love it or hate it. If you hate shopping, do you feel like you're broken? Is something wrong with you? Aren't all women supposed to love to shop? We have been surprised to find that most women

You can also feel exhausted when you shop for hours and nothing seems to fit or isn't the right color. Remember to always shop when you're in a good mood and with your hair and makeup done. We assure you, you'll be more successful in finding things you love.

dislike shopping. Shopping can be exhausting and exhilarating all at the same time. You can be so excited and energized when you find an amazing article of clothing or a pair of shoes at a screaming good deal.

Remember, it's all about how you feel. When you take time to select clothes that you feel fabulous in, and that will make you feel better about yourself, think about you. How do you feel when you purchase a new outfit and wear it for the first time? Aren't you worth the time and money to feel fabulous? You are a beautiful woman and should always celebrate you.

## Bonnie Moehle ~ life balancing coach and author talks about releasing the guilt.

Guilt is a useless emotion. We do feel guilt because we believe it shows that we care, that we have remorse or that we feel ashamed of what we've done. Sometimes, we do feel guilt because we feel that being hard on ourselves is what we deserve. Regardless of the reason for our guilt, it does not and will not make us healthier as people, nor will it erase what has already been done. Punishing ourselves with guilt does not change anything. It does, however, lower our energy and make us feel unhappy. How can we enjoy our choices if we are mired in guilt?

Guilt is a form of self-abuse, regret, and shame where we scold ourselves in an effort to feel worthwhile or to show that we care. The problem is that the feelings we are seeking through guilt just don't come to be. Guilt will not make us better! Why? Because every thought that we have about ourselves translates directly into the way we perceive, react, and behave. In other words, what we focus on becomes our behaviors, reactions, and experiences. Focusing on our faults causes emotionally painful behaviors, such as the perception that people are judging us, defensiveness, the setting of unhealthy boundaries, taking the words and actions of others personally, and depriving ourselves of the pleasures of life. When we make it a practice to focus on our strengths, these perceptions and behaviors will fall away and we begin to treat both ourselves and others with a greater deal of love and respect.

Feeling guilty about taking care of ourselves is very prevalent today. As parents, we feel guilty about a night out on the town or a vacation without the kids. As children of elderly parents, we feel guilty about never doing enough. As coworkers, we feel guilty for taking a day off from work, and, of course, we really feel terrible when we indulge ourselves with something nice. Treating ourselves to something nice every now and then can be very beneficial. Yes, there are those with unhealthy spending habits, or those who use shopping as a distraction from their emotions. But for those of us who spend responsibly, a treat to ourselves is a symbol of self-worth and self-respect. It is a statement that says, *"I'm worth it and I deserve it."* Feeling guilty about our acquisitions is a demonstration of a lack of self-respect and a feeling of unworthiness. We are worthy!

We can let go of guilt by beginning a healthy practice of appreciating ourselves daily. We can be more aware of all of the smart, helpful, creative, and kind things we do all of the time because they are already a part of who we are. We just forgot to notice. We can look into the mirror each morning and tell ourselves what we love about ourselves. We can live more in the present moment, enjoying where we are rather than projecting into the past or the future. When we let go of a destructive emotions such as guilt, we have clarity. We are more capable of making smart choices and we enjoy life more fully.

# ~ Bonnie

## HOW DOES YOUR CLOSET MAKE YOU FEEL?

Having a clean, clutter free and organized closet will make you feel great. Does your environment reflect your inner self? Let's get organized.

**Now that you've purged your wardrobe, it will be a breeze to organize.**

It may have looked like a thrift store before but you're about to create a designer boutique right in your own closet.

When things are just hung up randomly, it will look messy. However, if you hang clothes by color and type, you will love to open your closet door. You can double hang your rods and place your tops on the top rod and bottoms on the lower rack. If your closet doesn't currently have double rods, you can add one yourself very easily.

## GET SOME REALLY NICE QUALITY HANGERS.

I love wooden hangers, but if you're short on space, Brenda Spangrud with SORTED Organizing recommends the black velvet slim hangers. They miraculously create more space in your closet. You can also create your own vertical rod and hang a chain from an "s" hook.

If you have shelving space, this is a great place to store items like purses and sweaters.

Brenda Spangrud ~ professional organizer and speaker talks about organizing your closet.

## THREE STEPS TO AN ORGANIZED CLOSET

Does your closet look more like a thrift store than a boutique? If so, chances are good that those "feel good" "look great" outfits aren't jumping out at you saying "pick me" "pick me." Instead, you probably feel overwhelmed and lost when you open your closet doors and experience what I call "closet confusion."

Follow these three organizing tips to avoid closet confusion and start your mornings off on the right foot...and with the right outfit.

1. <u>Know what's in there</u>: Purge, purge, then RUTHLESSLY purge! Most people collect clothes like they collect photographs. They can head in to the closet and start picking out pieces and

telling the stories behind each piece. Ah...remember when..? Your closet is a place to store the clothes you DO WEAR, not an archive to accumulate mementos!

By having items that no longer make you feel or look great crammed within your current wardrobe options, you literally do have a closet full of clothes and nothing to wear! Similar to finding a needle in a haystack.

Create a fresh start and weed out all those items that you don't currently wear.  Any items you feel a need to hold on to for sentimental reasons, take off the hanger and fold them in to a nice storage bin that can be placed in a far corner on the floor or up high out of your valuable space.

Getting ready in the morning will be a breeze if your only choices are those that suit you.

## 2. What's Hot and What's Not Reference Book: If

your closet resembles a boutique and you find yourself overwhelmed by too many choices, or you find you are wearing the same outfit over and over again, consider creating a "What's Hot" reference book.  This can be your go-to memory jogger of some outfit combinations you may have forgot about.  This is very helpful if you experience morning brain fog and aren't your most creative self first thing in the morning.

This book can be as simple as a journal that you make notes within and place stars next to. For instance: Black lacy top, white jeans, black sling backs, chunky silver necklace, and hoop earrings. Received compliments all day—five stars.  Or you can take picture of yourself in a mirror and tape the pictures within pages of a notebook.

Keep this book tucked on a shelf in the closet for easy reference. The key is to keep it simple and easy to use.

## 3. <u>Organize your clothes for Visual Pairing</u>: There are

many different methods in which to organize your closet. Some of the most common ways are by color (all green items hang together, etc.), by season (winter, spring, summer, or fall), by occasion (casual, work, or formal wear) or by item (short sleeves, long sleeves, pants, dresses, etc.).

You choose whichever method makes sense to you and makes your routine easier. However, my favorite method and the method of which I encourage my clients to use is the "by item" method.

By organizing your clothes and keeping like items together, you'll have clean visual lines in which to spot a particular piece of clothing and items which are kept within seasons automatically.

When choosing an outfit, most people start off with checking in first with what they're in the mood to wear, then looking for the items that support that mood. For instance, I'm feeling flirty or feminine today and want to wear a skirt or dress. Then I check in with what the temperature will be like that day and decided it will be cool. So, I go to the section with my dresses and check to see if any of them appeal to me. If not, I then browse my skirts. If I choose a skirt, then choosing a top is next. If all my short sleeve tops are lined up together and all my and cardigan sweaters are together, my selections are easy to see and my choices take less time to make. If your closet is divided with top hanging rods and bottom hanging rods, try and hang your tops on the top handing rods and pants or skirts on bottom hanging rods. This will make visual pairing that much easier.

Closets come in many different shapes and sizes, just like their owners. But no matter what size of closet you have, chances are good that you're saying you don't have enough space. An entire book could be devoted to the different products and solutions to maximize every square inch within the closet. What I'd like to share with you is this simple rule: if you see wall, you have an opportunity for more space.

If you utilize the method of hanging like items together, you'll open up storage space on the floor underneath your short hanging items, such as your shirts or skirts. Utilize this storage space by stacking on the floor, clear totes filled with purses or folded jeans. If your closet has accordion doors, an open wall is a perfect place to hang a "behind the door" shoe pocket organizer filled with scarves, ties, belts, hats, bras, etc. If there's empty space, consider it a storage opportunity and be creative with your storage solutions so that you can maximize storage.

Closet space is one of the prime storage spaces in a home. Don't treat your clothes' closet like a dumping ground for whatever needs stored. Create storage solutions with a defined purpose that are easy to use. The easier the systems are to use, the more likely you are to maintain them.

## ~ Brenda

## Thoughts to Reflect

1.  Always be aware of current fashion and styles. Be in the present.
2.  Review magazines and websites on fashion and style.
3.  Be conscious of "your" fashion style.
4.  Don't get stuck in a style rut.
5.  Review and purge your wardrobe a minimum of twice a year when the seasons change.
6.  Don't keep things that no longer serve you.
7.  Take a wing woman with you when shopping.
8.  Experiment with different combinations.
9.  Above all else, have fun! Fashion should be fun and make you feel fabulous!
10. And take your hair out of that damn ponytail!

Stylishly Yours,

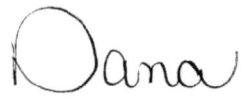

To order additional copies of this book:
www.doesthisponytail.com

To book Dana Lam and/or Emily Couch
as the speaker at your next event:
info@doesthisponytail.com

To hire Dana as your personal image
consultant:
dana@doesthisponytail.com

Also By Dana Lam

**5 Weeks to Fabulous**
A 5 week image and style tele-class
www.5weekstofabulous.com